Dealing with Your Time and Stress

An Exhaustive Aide

Stephen Rowling

Dealing with Your Time and Stress

An Exhaustive Aide

Jerry Colbert

3. Seek Help When Needed

4. Keep Learning

5. Celebrate Progress

Introduction

In our fast-paced, ever-changing world, the ability to effectively manage time and stress is not just a valuable skill; it is the foundation upon which we build our journey to a happier, more balanced life. The demands of our personal and professional lives can often seem overwhelming, leaving us in a perpetual battle against time and the physical and emotional toll of stress.

Yet, within the realm of these challenges lies the power to transform our lives. The journey to mastering time and stress is a quest for self-improvement, resilience, and well-being. It is a journey that can lead us to a place where we are not merely surviving but thriving, where each day is filled with purpose, productivity, and inner peace.

This book, "Dealing with Your Time and Stress: A Broad Aide," is your confided-in sidekick on this groundbreaking excursion. Here, we will delve deep into the art and science of time management and stress reduction, exploring a wealth of strategies, techniques, and insights that will empower you to regain control of your life. Whether you seek to enhance your productivity, improve your work-life balance, or simply find more joy in your daily existence, the wisdom within these pages will light your path.

As we embark on this adventure together, we will explore the roots of time-related stress and its emotional toll. We will uncover the secrets of effective time management, guiding you toward practices that make the most of your precious hours. We will shine a light on the sources of stress, from workplace demands to personal life challenges, offering invaluable insights into managing and mitigating its impact.

But this journey is not just about the external forces that shape our lives. It is equally about the internal landscapes of our minds and hearts. We will delve into the realms of self-care, resilience, and the power of mindfulness, learning how to nurture our emotional well-being and build inner strength.

Throughout this book, you will find practical exercises, real-life examples, and expert guidance that bridge the gap between theory and action. It is not enough to understand time and stress; we must apply this knowledge to create real, lasting change. Whether you are a professional seeking greater productivity, a parent striving for a better work-life balance, or an individual yearning for a more fulfilling existence, this book is tailored to meet you where you are and assist you with arriving at your objectives.

Together, we will explore the importance of balance, the value of self-assessment, and the significance of lifelong learning. This is not just a book; it is a roadmap to a more harmonious, empowered life.

So, as we turn the first page of this comprehensive guide, remember that you hold the pen to your own story. Your journey to mastering time and stress is a testament to your commitment to a life of balance and well-being. Let us embark on this transformational voyage, where each chapter is an opportunity for growth, and each page brings you closer to a life lived on your terms.

Chapter 1
Setting Priorities

Introduction

Time is a finite resource, and how you use it can significantly impact your productivity and overall well-being. Setting priorities is the foundational step in effective time management. In this chapter, we will explore the art of distinguishing between urgent and important tasks, creating a prioritized to-do list, and making strategic time investments.

1. Distinguishing Between Urgent and Important

The first step in setting priorities is understanding the difference between urgency and importance. Tasks can often be categorized into one of four quadrants:

Urgent and Important: These are tasks that demand immediate attention and are crucial to your goals. They often include crisis situations, important deadlines, or pressing matters that require your immediate focus.

Important but Not Urgent: These are tasks that are significant for your long-term goals but do not require immediate action. Models incorporate long-haul projects, self-awareness, and key preparation.

Urgent but Not Important: These are tasks that may demand your immediate attention but do not contribute significantly to your long-term goals. They often include interruptions, some emails, and minor issues that can be delegated or minimized.

Not Urgent and Not Important: These tasks should be minimized or eliminated from your routine. They are distractions and time-wasters that provide little to no value.

Understanding these distinctions allows you to focus on what truly matters. The key is to spend most of your time in the "Important but Not Urgent" quadrant, where you can proactively work on your long-term goals and reduce the number of undertakings that fall into the "Dire and Significant" class.

2. Creating a Prioritized To-Do List

Once you've identified the tasks that fall into the "Important but Not Urgent" quadrant, the next step is to create a prioritized to-do list. This list should be a dynamic document that helps you:

1. Recognize your most significant undertakings for the afternoon.

2. Allocate specific time slots for each task.

3. Eliminate or delegate less important tasks.

4. Stay flexible to adjust your list as the day progresses.

A prioritized to-do list keeps you organized, ensures that you tackle essential tasks first, and reduces the chances of feeling overwhelmed by a long list of unsorted tasks.

3. Making Strategic Time Investments

Time is a valuable currency, and how you invest it can significantly impact your productivity and success. Making strategic time investments involves:

1. Allocating time to your most important and challenging tasks when your energy and focus are at their peak.

2. Breaking larger tasks into smaller, more manageable steps to avoid feeling overwhelmed.

3. Eliminating time-wasting habits or activities that don't contribute to your goals.

4. Practicing time management techniques such as the Pomodoro Technique to boost productivity.

The way you invest your time determines the quality and efficiency of your work. By allocating your time strategically, you can accomplish more in less time and reduce the stress associated with unfinished tasks and looming deadlines.

Chapter 2
Planning and Goal Setting

Introduction

Effective time management begins with clear goals and a well-structured plan to achieve them. In this chapter, we will explore the process of planning and goal setting, which provides a roadmap for your daily, weekly, and long-term activities. This chapter will guide you in defining your goals, breaking them down into manageable tasks, and creating a flexible, realistic plan to reach your objectives.

1. Defining Short-Term and Long-Term Goals

Short-Term Goals: These are goals that you aim to achieve within a relatively brief time frame, usually within a few days to a few months. Short-term goals help you focus on immediate tasks and can serve as stepping stones to your long-term objectives. Examples include completing a work project, losing a specific amount of weight, or learning a new skill.

Long-Term Goals: **Long-term goals have a more extended time horizon, often spanning several months to several years. They provide a broader perspective and define the overall direction you want to move in life. Examples include achieving career advancement, running a marathon, or building financial security for retirement.**

2. Breaking Goals into Manageable Tasks

Long-term goals can often feel overwhelming. Breaking them down into smaller, manageable tasks makes them more achievable. This process involves:

Defining Milestones: **Identify key milestones or checkpoints that will mark your progress toward the long-term goal. For instance, if your long-term goal is to write a novel, your milestones could include completing each chapter.**

Creating Task Lists: **Once you've established milestones, create task lists for each one. These task lists will become your daily and weekly to-do lists. This approach** allows you to focus on completing smaller tasks, making the bigger goal less daunting.

Setting Deadlines: **Assign deadlines to each task or milestone. This creates a sense of urgency and commitment, helping you stay on track and motivated.**

3. Creating a Realistic Plan

Creating a plan involves setting a clear path to achieving your goals. This is the way to make a sensible arrangement:

Focus on Your Objectives: **Not all objectives are similarly significant. Identify your top priorities and allocate more resources, time, and energy to them.**

Allocate Time and Resources: **Determine how much time and what resources are needed for each task and milestone. Be realistic about what you can accomplish in the available time frame.**

Adaptability and Flexibility: **Life is unpredictable, and plans may need adjustments. Being flexible allows you to adapt to unforeseen circumstances without losing sight of your goals.**

Track Progress: **Regularly review your plan and your progress. Use this information to make necessary adjustments and stay on course.**

A well-structured plan not only gives you direction but also boosts your motivation. As you achieve each milestone and complete tasks, you'll experience a sense of accomplishment that drives you to continue.

Chapter 3
Time-Blocking and Scheduling

Introduction

Time-blocking and scheduling are essential tools for effective time management. They allow you to allocate your time efficiently, ensuring that you have dedicated slots for specific tasks and activities. In this chapter, we will explore the techniques of time-blocking, creating daily and weekly schedules, and achieving a balance between structure and flexibility in your time management approach.

1. Using Time Blocks for Efficient Task Management

What Is Time-Blocking? Time-blocking is a method of allocating specific time blocks to tasks and activities throughout the day. These blocks can range from 15 minutes to several hours, depending on the task's complexity and importance.

The Benefits of Time-Blocking: **Time-blocking offers** several benefits, including enhanced focus, increased productivity, and the ability to avoid multitasking. It allows you to dedicate your full attention to a single task, which often leads to better results.

Creating Time Blocks: **Begin by identifying your top** priorities for the day. Assign specific time blocks to these tasks and allocate your most productive times to your most important work. Avoid overloading your schedule with tasks and leave buffer times for breaks and unexpected interruptions.

2. Crafting Daily and Weekly Schedules

Daily Schedules: **A daily schedule outlines your activities** for a specific day. It typically includes your work hours, appointments, time-blocked tasks, and personal commitments. Having a daily schedule keeps you on track and helps you make the most of each day.

Weekly Schedules: **A weekly schedule provides an** overview of your entire week. It allows you to plan for longer-term objectives, such as setting aside time for project work, exercise, or family activities. Creating a weekly schedule ensures that you allocate time for both immediate tasks and those that contribute to your long-term goals.

3. Balancing Rigidity and Flexibility

The Importance of Flexibility: **While structure is crucial for effective time management, it's equally important to remain flexible. Life is unpredictable, and unexpected events can disrupt your schedule. Accept that some level of flexibility is necessary to adapt to changing circumstances.**

Adjusting Your Schedule: **When unexpected interruptions occur or your priorities shift, be prepared to adjust your schedule. This might involve rescheduling tasks, rearranging time blocks, or delegating certain responsibilities.**

The Art of Saying No: **Part of managing your schedule effectively is learning to say no to tasks or commitments that don't align with your priorities. This permits you to safeguard your time and spotlight on the main thing.**

Conclusion

Time-blocking and scheduling are powerful tools for managing your time efficiently. By allocating specific time blocks to tasks and activities, you can enhance your focus and productivity. Daily and weekly schedules provide a roadmap for your activities, ensuring that you allocate time for immediate tasks and those that contribute to your long-term goals.

Balancing structure and flexibility in your schedule is key to effective time management. Recognize that while planning is important, life is unpredictable, and adjustments are sometimes necessary. Being flexible allows you to adapt to changing circumstances without feeling overwhelmed. In the upcoming chapters, we will explore additional time management techniques that complement these scheduling strategies.

Chapter 4
Delegation and Outsourcing

Introduction

Delegation and outsourcing are vital strategies in time management. Recognizing that you don't have to do everything yourself allows you to focus your time and energy on your most critical tasks. In this chapter, we will delve into the process of identifying tasks suitable for delegation, selecting reliable individuals or services for delegation, and establishing clear and effective communication for successful outsourcing.

1. Identifying Delegatable Tasks

The first step in effective delegation is recognizing which tasks can be delegated. Consider the following factors:

Skill Requirement: Tasks that do not require your unique skills or expertise are prime candidates for delegation. These tasks can often be performed by others competently.

Time-Intensity: Tasks that are time-intensive but do not necessarily demand your direct involvement are also suitable for delegation. Examples include data entry, research, or routine administrative work.

Routine and Repetitive Tasks: Tasks that are repetitive and can be standardized are typically good choices for delegation. These tasks can often be handled more efficiently by others.

2. Selecting Reliable Delegation Partners

Once you've identified tasks suitable for delegation, the next step is to choose the right individuals or services for the job. Consider the following criteria:

Competence: Ensure that the person or service you delegate to has the necessary skills and knowledge to perform the task effectively.

Trustworthiness: Trust is paramount in delegation. You should have confidence that the person or service you delegate to will complete the task as expected.

Communication Skills: **Effective communication is key.** Clear and open communication with your delegation partner helps ensure that expectations are well-defined and understood.

3. Effective Communication for Delegation

Successful delegation hinges on effective communication. To ensure that tasks are executed as intended, consider the following communication strategies:

Clear Instructions: Provide comprehensive instructions, including task details, deadlines, and desired outcomes. Ensure that your delegation partner fully understands what is expected.

Check-ins: **Establish a system for regular check-ins and progress updates. This allows you to monitor the task's status and address any questions or issues that arise.**

Feedback and Accountability: **Create a feedback loop** that allows for constructive feedback and accountability.

This encourages quality work and continuous improvement.

Conclusion

Delegation and outsourcing are powerful techniques that allow you to focus your time and energy on tasks that truly require your expertise and attention. By identifying tasks suitable for delegation, selecting reliable individuals or services, and maintaining effective communication, you can improve your time management significantly. Delegation not only helps you free up time but also fosters collaboration and skill development among your team or partners.

In the subsequent chapters, we will explore additional time management strategies and techniques that complement delegation and outsourcing, helping you optimize your productivity and reduce stress.

Chapter 5
Understanding Stress

Introduction

Stress is an inherent part of life, and understanding it is the first step in managing it effectively. This chapter delves into the sources of stress, its physical and emotional impact, and the distinction between beneficial and harmful stress.

1. Recognizing Stress Sources

Stress can stem from various sources, including:

Workplace Stress: Demands, deadlines, and conflicts in the workplace.

Personal Life Stress: Family issues, relationships, or financial concerns.

Health-Related Stress: Illness, injuries, or chronic health conditions.

Environmental Stress: External factors such as noise, traffic, or living conditions.

Understanding the sources of your stress is crucial in addressing them effectively. By identifying the root causes, you can develop targeted strategies to manage or reduce stress.

2. Understanding the Physical and Emotional Impact

Stress can manifest physically and emotionally, affecting your body and mind. Common physical symptoms of stress include:

Muscle tension

Rapid heartbeat

Headaches

Digestive issues

Fatigue

Emotionally, stress can lead to:

Anxiety

Irritability

Mood swings

Difficulty concentrating

Feeling overwhelmed

Recognizing these physical and emotional signs of stress can help you identify when you're under stress and take proactive steps to manage it.

3. The Fine Line Between Beneficial and Harmful Stress

Not all stress is bad. Some stress, known as eustress, is beneficial and can enhance your performance. For example, the stress associated with a challenging project can motivate you to excel. However, excessive or chronic stress, known as distress, can have harmful effects on your physical and mental well-being.

Understanding the balance between beneficial and harmful stress is crucial. It helps you harness the positive aspects of stress while developing strategies to mitigate its negative impact.

Conclusion

Stress is a general occurrence, but you let it control your life. By recognizing the sources of stress, understanding its physical and emotional impact, and distinguishing between beneficial and harmful stress, you can take the first step in effective stress management.

Chapter 6
Stress Reduction Techniques

Introduction

Now that we've explored the sources and impact of stress, it's time to delve into practical stress reduction techniques. This chapter will guide you through a variety of strategies to manage and alleviate stress, including relaxation techniques, exercise, and the importance of quality sleep.

1. Relaxation Techniques

Relaxation techniques are powerful tools for reducing stress and promoting mental well-being. Some effective relaxation techniques include:

Deep Breathing: Deep, slow, and controlled breathing helps calm the nervous system, reduce tension, and lower stress levels. Practice deep breathing exercises to manage stress when it arises.

Meditation and Mindfulness: These practices encourage living in the present moment and promoting inner peace. Regular meditation and mindfulness exercises can reduce anxiety and stress.

Progressive Muscle Relaxation: This technique involves progressively tensing and relaxing different muscle groups, helping release physical tension.

Visualization: Guided imagery and visualization exercises can transport you to a peaceful and stress-free mental space, reducing anxiety and promoting relaxation.

2. Exercise and Stress Reduction

Physical activity is a natural stress reliever. Engaging in regular exercise can:

Release Endorphins: Exercise stimulates the release of endorphins, natural mood elevators that reduce stress and boost overall well-being.

Promote Better Sleep: **A consistent exercise routine can improve the quality of your sleep, which is essential for stress management.**

Provide a Sense of Control: **Regular exercise can give you a sense of control over your body and health, which can help reduce stress associated with feeling powerless.**

3. The Importance of Quality Sleep

Adequate, restorative sleep is essential for stress management. When you're well-rested, you're better equipped to cope with stress. To improve the quality of your sleep:

Establish a Sleep Routine: **Go to bed and wake up at the same times every day, even on weekends.**

Create a Relaxing Bedtime Ritual: **Engage in calming activities before sleep, such as reading, listening to soothing music, or taking a warm bath.**

Ensure a Comfortable Sleep Environment: **Your bedroom should be dark, cool, and quiet, with a comfortable mattress and pillows.**

Conclusion

Effective stress management requires a multifaceted approach, and relaxation techniques, exercise, and quality sleep play significant roles in reducing stress and enhancing well-being. By incorporating these strategies into your daily routine, you can better cope with stress and improve your overall mental and physical health.

Chapter 7
Time for Self-Care

Introduction

Self-care is the practice of taking deliberate steps to nurture your physical, emotional, and mental well-being. In this chapter, we will explore the importance of self-care, the activities that can promote it, and the significance of setting boundaries to protect your time.

1. Prioritizing Activities That Bring Joy

Self-care is about doing things that make you happy and promote a sense of well-being. This includes activities like:

Hobbies: Engaging in hobbies you're passionate about, whether it's painting, playing a musical instrument, gardening, or any other creative pursuit.

Spending Time in Nature: Nature has a calming effect and spending time outdoors can reduce stress. Activities like hiking, biking, or simply taking a walk in a park can be rejuvenating.

Social Connection: Nurturing relationships with friends and family. Significant social associations can offer profound help and lessen sensations of seclusion.

2. Setting Boundaries for Personal Time

Setting boundaries is essential to protect your time and self-care practices. It involves:

Saying No: Learning to decline additional commitments when your schedule is already full. Focusing on your prosperity isn't egotistical; it's important.

Time Management: Allocating specific time blocks in your schedule for self-care activities. Treat these meetings with a similar degree of significance as work gatherings.

Disconnecting: Taking breaks from technology and work-related tasks. Unplugging from devices and work emails allows your mind to rest and recover.

3. Practicing Self-Compassion and Mindfulness

Self-sympathy includes treating yourself with consideration and understanding, particularly during testing times. Mindfulness, on the other hand, is the practice of being present at the moment without judgment. These practices can:

Reduce self-criticism and negative self-talk.

Promote emotional resilience.

Enhance your overall sense of well-being.

Conclusion

Self-care is not a luxury; it's a necessity for maintaining your physical and mental health. Prioritizing activities that bring joy, setting boundaries to protect your time, and practicing self-compassion and mindfulness are essential components of self-care.

In the chapters ahead, we will explore problem-solving and coping techniques, the balance between work and personal life, and the importance of evaluating your progress. These strategies will further contribute to your overall stress management and self-care practices.

Chapter 8
Problem-Solving and Coping

Introduction

Life inevitably presents challenges and problems, and how you address them can significantly impact your stress levels. This chapter focuses on identifying sources of stress, effective problem-solving techniques, and developing healthy coping mechanisms.

1. Identifying Sources of Stress and Their Root Causes

To effectively manage stress, you must first understand its sources. This involves:

Self-Reflection: Take time to reflect on the sources of your stress. Are they primarily work-related, personal, or health-related? Understanding the specific triggers can help you address them more effectively.

Root Cause Analysis: **Consider what underlies the sources of your stress. For example, if work-related deadlines cause stress, is it due to excessive workload, a lack of time management, or unrealistic expectations?**

Recognizing Patterns: **Identifying recurring sources of stress allows you to develop targeted strategies for prevention or resolution.**

2. Problem-Solving Techniques

Effective problem-solving is essential in stress management. Some problem-solving techniques include:

Characterize the Issue: **Obviously, lucid the issue you're confronting. Be specific about what needs to be addressed.**

Brainstorm Solutions: **Generate multiple potential solutions, without judgment. Quantity is more important than quality in this stage.**

Evaluate Solutions: **Assess each potential solution based on its feasibility and potential effectiveness.**

Implement and Evaluate: **Once you've chosen a solution, put it into action and evaluate its impact. If it doesn't work, return to the brainstorming phase.**

3. Developing Healthy Coping Mechanisms

Coping mechanisms are strategies or behaviors that help you deal with stress. Healthy coping mechanisms include:

Exercise: **Physical activity releases endorphins, reduces stress, and provides a healthy outlet for pent-up tension.**

Mindfulness and Meditation: **These practices can help you stay grounded and reduce the emotional impact of stressors.**

Seeking Support: **Talking to a friend, family member, or mental health professional can provide emotional support and a fresh perspective.**

Time Management: **Effective time management and organization can reduce stress associated with deadlines and commitments.**

Conclusion

Understanding the sources of your stress, developing problem-solving skills, and adopting healthy coping mechanisms are key components of effective stress management. By addressing problems proactively and implementing healthy strategies, you can reduce the impact of stress on your life.

Chapter 9
Creating a Balanced Life

Introduction

Balancing the demands of work, personal life, and self-care is crucial for effective stress management. In this chapter, we will explore the concept of work-life balance, strategies for maintaining a healthy lifestyle, and the importance of communication in safeguarding your well-being.

1. The Importance of Work-Life Balance

Work-life balance refers to the equilibrium between the time and energy you invest in your professional and personal life. It is essential for stress management for several reasons:

Preventing Burnout: Excessive focus on work at the expense of personal life can lead to burnout, chronic stress, and decreased productivity.

Enhancing Well-Being: Spending quality time with family and engaging in personal interests contributes to your overall well-being and happiness.

Improved Mental Health: Achieving work-life balance reduces the risk of stress-related mental health issues, such as anxiety and depression.

2. Strategies for Maintaining a Healthy Lifestyle

Maintaining a healthy lifestyle is integral to stress management. Key strategies include:

Exercise: Regular physical activity not only reduces stress but also improves overall health.

Nutrition: A well-balanced diet provides the necessary nutrients for both physical and mental health.

Sleep: Prioritizing quality sleep ensures that you have the energy and mental clarity to cope with stress effectively.

Social Connections: **Cultivating and maintaining healthy relationships contributes to your overall well-being and provides emotional support.**

3. Communicating Your Needs

Effective communication is vital in maintaining work-life balance. This includes:

Setting Boundaries: **Clearly communicate your boundaries to colleagues, supervisors, and family members. Let them know when you are unavailable for work-related tasks and when you need personal time.**

Asking for Support: **Don't hesitate to ask for help or support when you're feeling overwhelmed. Communicating your needs allows your support network to assist you in times of high stress.**

Expressing Your Feelings: **Share your emotions and stressors with a trusted friend or family member. Often, voicing your concerns can provide relief and a fresh perspective.**

Conclusion

Creating a balanced life by embracing work-life balance, maintaining a healthy lifestyle, and effective communication are essential components of stress management. These strategies not only help reduce the impact of stress but also contribute to your overall well-being and happiness.

Chapter 10
Staying Consistent

Introduction

Consistency is a powerful force in time and stress management. This chapter delves into the significance of maintaining consistency in your daily routines, how it can enhance your productivity, and how to adapt to life changes while preserving healthy habits.

1. The Power of Consistency

Consistency in your daily routines and habits can lead to several benefits in time and stress management:

Predictability: Knowing what to expect from your daily routines reduces uncertainty and, subsequently, stress.

Improved Productivity: Consistency allows you to build momentum and accomplish tasks more efficiently.

Reduced Decision Fatigue: **Routines eliminate the need to make countless decisions about mundane tasks, preserving your mental energy for more important matters.**

2. Adapting to Life Changes and Evolutions

Life is dynamic, and your routines may need adjustment to accommodate changes. Key considerations include:

Flexibility: **While consistency is valuable, you must also remain adaptable. When life circumstances change, be open to modifying your routines to suit your new reality.**

Prioritization: **Identify your essential habits and routines, and make sure they remain consistent, even as other aspects of your life shift.**

Stress Management in Transitions: **Major life transitions, such as a new job, family changes, or relocation, can be highly stressful. Recognize the added stress in these situations and make self-care a priority.**

3. Maintaining Healthy Routines

Consistency in maintaining healthy routines, such as exercise, sleep, and self-care, is particularly crucial for stress management. Ensure that these routines remain a constant, even when other aspects of your life change.

Conclusion

Consistency in your daily routines is a cornerstone of effective time and stress management. While maintaining healthy habits is essential, it's equally important to adapt to life changes while preserving your well-being. By finding the right balance between consistency and adaptability, you can navigate life's ups and downs more effectively and manage stress with resilience.

Chapter 11
Seeking Professional Help

Introduction

Sometimes, despite our best efforts, stress can become overwhelming, and it may be necessary to seek professional assistance. This chapter discusses when and how to seek help, the various professionals who can provide support, and the benefits of therapy in stress management.

1. Recognizing the Need for Professional Help

It's important to recognize when the stress you're experiencing has become unmanageable and is significantly impacting your life. Signs that might show a requirement for proficient assistance include:

Persistent Anxiety or Depression: If you're experiencing ongoing feelings of anxiety or depression that interfere with your daily life.

Chronic Stress: **When stress becomes chronic, leading to health issues or affecting your overall well-being.**

Inability to Cope: **If you're struggling to cope with stress or facing overwhelming life changes.**

Interference with Work or Relationships: **When stress negatively affects your job performance or relationships with others.**

2. Professionals Who Can Provide Support

There are various professionals who can help you manage stress effectively:

Therapists and Counselors: **These professionals specialize in helping individuals cope with mental health challenges, stress, and personal difficulties.**

Psychiatrists: **Psychiatrists are medical doctors who can prescribe medication if necessary for managing stress and related mental health issues.**

Support Groups: **Participating in support groups can provide a sense of community and shared experiences, allowing you to learn from others facing similar challenges.**

3. The Benefits of Therapy

Therapy, also known as counseling or psychotherapy, is an effective way to manage and reduce stress. Benefits of therapy include:

Learning Coping Strategies: **Therapists can teach you practical strategies for dealing with stress and its impact.**

Emotional Support: **Having a safe, confidential space to discuss your concerns and emotions can provide immense relief.**

Identifying Underlying Issues: **Therapy can help you uncover and address the root causes of your stress.**

Conclusion

Seeking professional help is a valid and valuable step in managing and reducing stress. Recognizing when it's necessary, understanding the types of professionals available, and appreciating the benefits of therapy can empower you to navigate stressful situations more effectively.

Chapter 12
Building Resilience

Introduction

Resilience is the capacity to adjust to pressure and affliction. In this chapter, we will explore the concept of resilience, strategies to build and strengthen it, and how resilience contributes to effective stress management.

1. Understanding Resilience

Resilience is not just about enduring stress but thriving despite it. It involves:

Adaptability: The capacity to adjust and cope with changes and challenges effectively.

Emotional Strength: The ability to manage emotions, maintain a positive outlook, and bounce back from setbacks.

Problem-Solving Skills: The skill to navigate challenges and find solutions.

2. Strategies to Build Resilience

Resilience is a skill that can be developed and strengthened. Key strategies for building resilience include:

Cultivating a Support System: Building and maintaining a strong network of friends, family, and colleagues who provide emotional support.

Practicing Self-Care: Prioritizing self-care activities, maintaining healthy routines, and engaging in relaxation techniques to reduce stress.

Staying Positive: Fostering a positive outlook on life, even in challenging times, can improve your resilience.

Developing Problem-Solving Skills: Enhancing your ability to approach problems rationally and find effective solutions.

3. Resilience and Stress Management

Resilience and stress management are closely connected. When you are more resilient, you can:

Bounce Back: **Resilience allows you to recover more quickly from stress and adversity.**

Stay Proactive: **Resilient individuals are better at proactive stress management and problem-solving.**

Maintain Emotional Balance: **Resilience helps you keep emotional stability, even in stressful situations.**

Conclusion

Building resilience is a key factor in effective stress management. By developing the skills and strategies necessary to adapt to adversity and thrive under stress, you can significantly reduce the impact of stress on your life.

Chapter 13
Managing Technology's Impact

Introduction

Technology plays a significant role in our lives, both enhancing and complicating our time and stress management. This chapter explores the impact of technology on stress, strategies to manage it, and how to strike a healthy balance between technology use and well-being.

1. The Impact of Technology on Stress

Technology can contribute to stress in various ways, such as:

Information Overload: The constant stream of information and notifications can lead to feeling overwhelmed and anxious.

Digital Distractions: Technology can divert your attention, making it challenging to stay focused on important tasks.

Reduced Sleep Quality: Excessive screen time, especially before bed, can disrupt sleep patterns, leading to increased stress.

2. Strategies for Managing Technology-Related Stress

To manage technology's impact on your stress levels effectively, consider these strategies:

Digital Detox: Periodically disconnect from screens and digital devices. This can be done for a few hours each day or as a more extended break, such as a weekend.

Establish Boundaries: Set specific boundaries for technology use. For example, make "no-screen" times during the day.

Screen Time Tracking: **Utilize apps or features that track your screen time. This can help you become more aware of your usage patterns.**

Mindful Tech Use: **Practice mindful technology usage by being present and purposeful when engaging with digital devices.**

3. Striking a Healthy Balance

Striking a balance between the benefits of technology and its potential stress-inducing aspects is key. Consider:

Utilizing Productivity Apps: **Use technology to your advantage by exploring productivity apps and tools that can help you manage time more effectively.**

Limiting Social Media: **Be selective about your social media usage and ensure it contributes positively to your life.**

Engaging in Offline Activities: **Balance screen time with offline activities that promote well-being, such as exercise, hobbies, and social interactions.**

Conclusion

Technology is an integral part of modern life, and understanding its impact on stress is crucial. By implementing strategies to manage technology-related stress and striking a healthy balance between the benefits and drawbacks of technology, you can harness its advantages while reducing its negative impact on your stress levels.

Chapter 14
Evaluating Your Progress

Introduction

Evaluating your progress in stress management is crucial for ongoing improvement and well-being. In this chapter, we will explore the significance of self-assessment, how to track your progress, and the role of reflection in your stress management journey.

1. The Importance of Self-Assessment

Self-assessment is the process of reflecting on your stress management journey, recognizing your achievements, and identifying areas for improvement. It is vital because it:

Provides Clarity: Self-assessment helps you gain clarity on what strategies and techniques work best for you.

Promotes Accountability: **Regularly evaluating your progress holds you accountable for your well-being and stress management efforts.**

Encourages Adaptation: **Self-assessment allows you to adapt your approach as life circumstances change.**

2. Tracking Your Progress

To effectively evaluate your progress, consider the following:

Establish Clear Metrics: **Set specific metrics and goals for your stress management journey. This could include reducing stress levels, improving sleep quality, or increasing overall well-being.**

Use Tools and Journals: **Utilize stress-tracking apps, journals, or diaries to record your experiences and feelings. This will help you identify patterns and changes over time.**

Regular Check-Ins: **Schedule regular check-ins with yourself to reflect on your progress. Consider doing this weekly or monthly.**

3. The Role of Reflection

Reflection is a key component of self-assessment. It involves looking back on your experiences, decisions, and actions. In your stress management journey:

Celebrate Success: **Acknowledge and celebrate your achievements, no matter how small they may seem.**

Learn from Setbacks: **When you encounter setbacks or challenges, use them as opportunities for learning and growth.**

Adjust Your Approach: **If you identify strategies that are not working, be open to adjusting your approach and trying new techniques.**

Conclusion

Evaluating your progress in stress management is an ongoing and valuable process. By regularly assessing your journey, tracking your progress, and reflecting on your experiences, you can continue to improve your stress management skills and overall well-being.

Chapter 15
Sustaining Stress Management for Life

Introduction

Your stress management journey has been comprehensive, and this final chapter serves as a conclusion, offering guidance on sustaining the strategies you've learned for a lifetime of well-being. It emphasizes the importance of consistency, continuous learning, and adapting to life's ever-changing circumstances.

1. Consistency is Key

Consistency is at the heart of effective stress management. To sustain your progress, remember the following:

Maintain Healthy Routines: Keep up with the healthy habits you've developed, whether it's regular exercise, good nutrition, or relaxation techniques.

Set and Review Goals: **Continue to set specific goals for your stress management journey and regularly review your progress.**

Self-Assessment: **Consistently evaluate your stress management strategies to ensure they remain effective for your evolving life.**

2. The Value of Lifelong Learning

Learning about stress management is an ongoing process. As you move forward, consider:

Stay Informed: **Keep up with the latest research and information on stress management, self-care, and well-being.**

Explore New Techniques: **Be open to trying new stress management techniques and adapting your approach as new methods become available.**

Seek Professional Guidance: **If necessary, continue seeking professional help or counseling to navigate life's challenges effectively.**

3. Adapting to Life's Changes

Life is filled with changes, and your stress management strategies should adapt accordingly:

Recognize Life Transitions: **Major life events, such as career changes, family additions, or relocations, may require adjustments to your stress management techniques.**

Resilience and Adaptability: **Lean on the resilience you've built to adapt to new circumstances and stressors effectively.**

Maintain a Support System: **Continue nurturing your support network, as friends and family play a crucial role in your stress management journey.**

Conclusion

A Life of Balance and Well-Being

Your stress management journey is a lifelong commitment to your well-being. By prioritizing consistency, continuous learning, and adapting to life's changes, you can ensure that your stress management strategies remain effective and contribute to a fulfilling and stress-resilient life.

Your journey to effective stress management is a testament to your commitment to a happier, healthier, and more balanced life. May it serve as a reminder that your well-being is a priority worth every effort.

Your journey through this comprehensive guide on managing time and stress has equipped you with a treasure trove of knowledge, strategies, and techniques to lead a balanced and fulfilling life. As you embark on this new chapter, remember that your well-being is a priority, and the skills you've acquired will be your compass.

1. Embrace Balance

Strive to maintain equilibrium in all aspects of your life, whether it's work and personal life, technology use and offline activities, or consistency and adaptation. Balance is the foundation of effective stress management.

2. Prioritize Self-Care

Never underestimate the power of self-care. Engage in activities that bring you joy, practice mindfulness, and protect your personal time with healthy boundaries.

3. Seek Help When Needed

Recognize that seeking professional help is a courageous step in managing your well-being. If you find yourself in need of assistance, don't hesitate to reach out to therapists, counselors, or support groups.

4. Keep Learning

The journey of stress management is ongoing. Continue to educate yourself, explore new techniques, and remain open to adapting your strategies as life unfolds.

5. Celebrate Progress

Pause for a minute to recognize your accomplishments, regardless of how little. Celebrate your successes and use setbacks as stepping stones to growth.

Your dedication to managing time and stress is an investment in a happier, healthier life. As you apply these strategies, you'll find that you have the power to not only reduce stress but also enhance your overall well-being.

With this knowledge, you are now better equipped to navigate the complexities of life, make the most of your time, and lead a life filled with balance and well-being. Remember that this is a journey, and your commitment to self-improvement is a gift that keeps on giving.

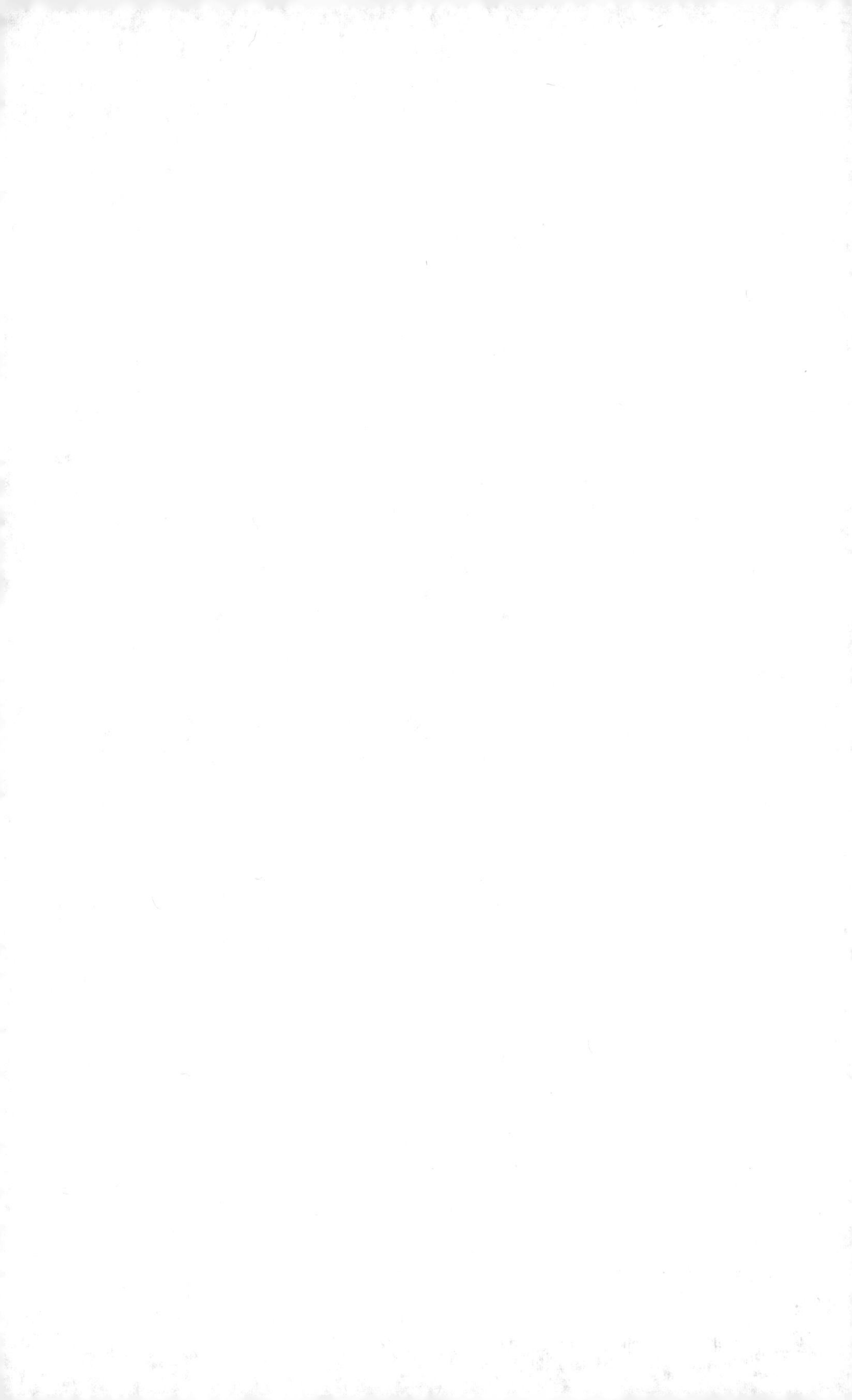

www.ingramcontent.com/pod-product-compliance
Lightning Source LLC
Chambersburg PA
CBHW061009260726
48661CB00005B/2126